MW01234562

Table of Contents

Introduction

Welcome to "Home Gym Mastery: Building Your Perfect Workout Space." I'm thrilled to have you on this journey to creating the ideal workout space right in the comfort of your home. There are so many benefits to having a home gym—convenience, privacy, and the ability to personalize your fitness routine, to name a few. Whether you're a seasoned fitness enthusiast or just starting out, having a dedicated space for exercise can really boost your motivation and consistency.

Let's dive into what this book is all about. We'll take you through every step of building your perfect home gym. We'll cover everything from assessing your available space to selecting the right equipment, designing an efficient layout, and personalizing the environment to match your preferences.

First things first, it's crucial to be clear about your fitness goals. Understanding what you want to achieve will help you make the best choices for your equipment and design. We'll talk about how to set effective fitness goals and develop a budget that works for you.

Once you have your goals and budget in place, we'll get into the fun part—designing your home gym. We'll look at principles of effective gym layout design and give you ideas on how to optimize your space. A motivating environment is key to keeping you engaged, so we'll also discuss ways to create a space that excites you.

When it comes to equipment, we've got you covered. We'll provide a comprehensive overview of essential home gym equipment, including cardio machines, strength training gear, and accessories. We'll help you weigh the pros and cons of each type, considering factors like space requirements, budget, and your specific fitness goals.

Beyond just selecting equipment, we'll guide you on how to organize your workout space for maximum functionality and convenience. We'll cover storage solutions, equipment placement, and multi-functional options to keep your gym tidy and efficient.

Creating an engaging atmosphere in your home gym is crucial. We'll explore ways to personalize your space, discussing strategies for enhancing the ambiance with decor, lighting, and motivational elements. Your workout space should uplift and energize you, making your workouts both physically and mentally rewarding.

Safety is paramount in any gym setting, and your home gym is no exception. We'll emphasize the importance of proper equipment assembly, maintenance, and injury prevention. Establishing a regular maintenance routine will ensure the longevity of your equipment and your safety during workouts.

Maximizing your workouts is essential to achieving your fitness goals. We'll provide techniques for designing versatile workouts that make the most of your available equipment and space. Adding variety and progression to your routines will help you avoid plateaus and keep your motivation high.

In today's digital age, technology can greatly enhance your home gym experience. We'll explore various options for integrating technology, such as fitness apps, virtual trainers, and interactive equipment features. Leveraging technology can help you track progress, stay motivated, and bring a new level of excitement to your workouts.

Finally, we'll discuss strategies for staying consistent and adapting your home gym setup and workout routine over time. We'll address common challenges like motivation slumps and time constraints. Being adaptable and making necessary adjustments will ensure that your home gym continues to meet your evolving fitness needs.

So, whether you're looking to build a small corner gym or a dedicated workout space, this book will serve as your ultimate guide to home gym mastery. Let's begin our journey towards creating the perfect workout sanctuary in your own home.

Chapter 1: Assessing Your Space

Let's get started on building your perfect home gym. The first step is all about assessing the available space you have. This chapter will guide you through evaluating your space and determining the best area for your workout haven.

Evaluating Available Space

Before you start transforming any room into a home gym, it's crucial to take a good look at the space you have. This means getting into the nitty-gritty details of the room's dimensions and layout. So, grab a tape measure and start noting down the measurements. Pay attention to any architectural features, like low ceilings, odd corners, or built-in shelves, that might impact your gym layout.

Another thing to think about is the natural light. How much sunlight does the room get? Natural light can make a huge difference in creating an energizing atmosphere. If your chosen space is a bit on the dark side, you might need to add some extra lighting fixtures. Adequate lighting isn't just for setting the mood; it's also essential for safety during your workouts.

Determining the Most Suitable Area for a Home Gym

Once you've got a clear picture of your available space, it's time to figure out which room in your house will best suit your fitness needs and preferences. Here are a few key factors to consider:

1. Noise Levels: Think about the noise you'll generate while working out. It's best to choose a room that's isolated from common living areas like bedrooms or the living room. This way, you won't disturb other household members with the sound of clanging weights or your favorite workout playlist.
2. Ventilation: Proper ventilation is a must for a comfortable workout environment. Look for a room with windows that allow for fresh air circulation. A well-ventilated space helps keep the air fresh and breathable, especially during intense workouts.
3. Flooring: The right flooring is essential for any home gym. You'll want something that provides cushioning and absorbs impact, like rubber or foam flooring. These options are great for

protecting your joints and reducing noise. Steer clear of carpeted areas, as they can make certain exercises difficult or even dangerous.

By carefully evaluating your space and considering factors like lighting, ventilation, and flooring, you'll be able to determine the most suitable area for your home gym. This foundation is key to creating an optimal workout environment that meets your fitness goals and preferences.

Now that you've assessed your space and determined the best area for your home gym, you're ready to move on to the next exciting step: setting your fitness goals and budget. But before we dive into that, take a moment to envision how you want your home gym to look and feel. Picture yourself in that space, working out and achieving your fitness goals. This vision will keep you motivated as we move forward on this journey together.

Chapter 2: Setting Goals and Budget

Hey again! Now that we've assessed your space, it's time to set some clear fitness goals and figure out a budget. This step is crucial because it helps you determine the design and equipment choices that will best suit your needs. So, let's dive in and get started on creating a home gym that truly works for you.

Establishing Clear Fitness Goals

The first thing you need to do when building your home gym is set clear fitness goals. These goals will guide your design and equipment choices. Take a moment to think about what you want to achieve with your workouts. Are you aiming to lose weight, build muscle, improve your cardiovascular fitness, or enhance your overall wellness? By defining your goals, you'll have a clear direction when it comes to selecting equipment and planning your workouts.

To establish clear fitness goals, ask yourself these questions:

1. What are my specific fitness objectives?

2. What activities or exercises do I enjoy the most?
3. How much time can I realistically commit to working out each week?
4. Do I prefer to focus on strength training, cardio exercises, or a combination of both?
5. Are there any specific milestones or events I am working towards?

Answering these questions will help you create a well-rounded and personalized fitness plan that aligns with your goals and preferences.

Aligning Goals with Design and Equipment Choices

Once you've set your fitness goals, it's time to align them with the design and equipment choices for your home gym. Here are some tips to help you make the best decisions:

1. Consider the space available: Take a good look at your available space and make sure it can accommodate the equipment you need to meet your goals. If space is limited, prioritize versatile and

multi-functional equipment that can be easily stored or folded when not in use.

2. Balance affordability with quality: Determine your budget and research equipment options that offer the best value for your money. While it's important to stick to a budget, remember that investing in high-quality equipment will provide greater durability and functionality in the long run.

3. Prioritize essential equipment: Identify the core equipment that aligns with your fitness goals. For example, if your primary focus is cardio fitness, consider investing in a treadmill or stationary bike. If strength training is your priority, choose a set of dumbbells or resistance bands.

4. Seek professional advice: Consult with fitness professionals or trainers who can provide guidance on the equipment and accessories that best suit your goals. They can offer insights into effective workout routines and recommend specific equipment based on your needs.

By aligning your goals with your design and equipment choices, you'll create a space that motivates and supports your fitness journey.

Strategies for Creating a Budget

Creating a budget for your home gym is an essential step to ensure that you make informed decisions about equipment purchases. Here are some strategies to help you balance affordability with quality and functionality:

1. Determine your overall budget: Start by establishing the maximum amount you can allocate to your home gym project. This will help you set realistic expectations and prioritize your spending.
2. Research equipment prices: Before making any purchases, research the prices of different types of equipment and compare them across various brands and retailers. Look for sales and discounts that may be available, and consider buying used equipment to save money.
3. Prioritize essential equipment: Identify the must-have equipment that aligns

with your goals and allocate a larger portion of your budget towards these items. Consider investing in high-quality, durable equipment that will withstand regular use.

4. Assess long-term costs: In addition to the initial equipment purchase, factor in any ongoing costs, such as maintenance, repairs, and replacement parts. This will help you make informed decisions about the longevity and value of the equipment you choose.

5. Consider alternatives and DIY options: Explore alternative options, such as resistance bands or bodyweight exercises, which can be more cost-effective than purchasing large and expensive equipment. Additionally, consider building your own equipment or repurposing items to save money.

6. Flexibility in budget allocation: Be prepared to adjust your budget allocation based on the prices and availability of equipment. Prioritize quality and functionality over quantity, and be willing to spend a little more for equipment that will provide a better workout experience.

By following these strategies, you can create a budget that allows you to achieve your fitness goals while being mindful of your financial resources. Remember, the ultimate goal is to create a home gym that is both effective and budget-friendly.

Now that you have established your fitness goals and created a reasonable budget, it's time to move on to the next chapter: Designing the Layout. This chapter will provide you with valuable insights on effectively organizing your home gym space for maximum functionality and aesthetics.

Chapter 3: Designing the Layout

Now that you've set your fitness goals and budget, it's time to design the layout of your home gym. A well-thought-out layout ensures efficient use of space, promotes safe movement, and creates a motivating environment to help you reach your fitness goals. Let's dive into the key principles of effective gym layout design and explore some ideas for optimizing your space.

Considerations for Traffic Flow

One of the most important aspects of designing your home gym layout is traffic flow. You want to make sure your gym allows for easy and safe movement between equipment. You definitely don't want to feel cramped or have to navigate through obstacles during your workouts. Here are some tips to help you optimize traffic flow:

1. Leave Enough Space Between Equipment: Ensure there is ample room between different pieces of equipment. This not only prevents potential clashes or accidents but also provides enough

space for you to move around and perform exercises comfortably.

2. Proximity of Cardio and Strength Training Areas: If your gym includes both cardio and strength training equipment, it's ideal to position them in separate areas or sections. This helps to minimize distractions and enables focused workouts.

3. Create Designated Workout Zones: Think about dividing your gym space into different zones for various types of exercises. For instance, have a specific area for cardio exercises, another for strength training, and maybe a designated stretching or yoga corner. This way, you can move seamlessly from one workout to another without constantly rearranging equipment.

Equipment Placement

The placement of your equipment is crucial to the overall layout and functionality of your home gym. Here are some tips for deciding where to place your equipment:

1. Prioritize Frequently Used Equipment: Place the equipment you use most

frequently within easy reach and in a prominent position. Items like dumbbells, resistance bands, and exercise mats should be readily accessible so you can incorporate them into your workouts without wasting time searching.

2. Plan for Efficient Workout Circuits: Arrange your equipment strategically to create efficient workout circuits. Group together equipment that is commonly used in combination or for supersets. This setup will make it easier to transition from one exercise to the next, saving you time and effort.

3. Utilize Vertical Space: If you have limited floor space, consider using vertical space to maximize your gym's capacity. Install sturdy shelves or racks to store smaller equipment or accessories like kettlebells or medicine balls. This not only saves space but also keeps your gym organized and clutter-free.

Accessibility

Ensuring the accessibility of your home gym is vital for a smooth workout experience. Here are a few considerations to keep in mind:

1. Clear Pathways: Make sure there are clear pathways leading to and from each piece of equipment, ensuring easy access without any obstructions. This will prevent tripping hazards and accidents.
2. Consider Height and Reach: Take into account the height and reach of each user when placing equipment. Consider adjustable equipment options to accommodate users of varying heights and abilities.
3. Incorporate Mirrors: Mirrors are a valuable addition to any gym. They not only create a sense of space but also allow you to check and maintain proper form during exercises. Place mirrors strategically to provide a full view of your workout area.

Creating a Balanced and Motivating Environment

Designing your home gym layout isn't just about practical considerations; it's also about creating a space that motivates and energizes you. Here are some ideas to help you achieve a balanced and motivating environment:

1. Utilize Natural Light: If possible, position your gym near a window to let in natural light. Natural light has a positive impact on mood and energy levels, creating a more inviting and motivating space.
2. Add Motivational Decor: Consider adding motivational quotes, posters, or images that inspire you to push harder and stay focused during your workouts. Personalize your gym with elements that reflect your fitness goals and aspirations.
3. Choose a Color Scheme Wisely: Colors can influence our emotions and energy levels. Opt for colors that promote energy, like vibrant hues or cool blues. Avoid colors that may have a calming effect, as you want your gym to be an energizing space.
4. Include Audiovisual Elements: Consider installing a speaker system or television in your gym to enhance your workout experience. Listening to energizing

music or watching workout videos can
keep you motivated and engaged.

By considering these principles of effective
layout design and implementing these ideas,
you can create a home gym that maximizes
space utilization, promotes efficient movement,
and motivates you to achieve your fitness
goals. Now that you've designed your gym
layout, let's move on to the next chapter:
Selecting Equipment.

Chapter 4: Selecting Equipment

Now that we've got a clear vision for your home gym layout, it's time to talk about equipment. Selecting the right gear is a crucial step in building your perfect workout space. In this chapter, we'll dive deep into the essential equipment for your home gym. We'll cover different types of cardio machines, strength training equipment, and useful accessories. Plus, we'll give you tips on how to choose the right equipment based on your fitness goals, available space, and budget.

Understanding Your Fitness Goals

Before we get into the specifics of equipment, it's important to have a clear understanding of your fitness goals. What are you hoping to achieve with your home workouts? Are you aiming to improve your cardiovascular endurance, build muscle, lose weight, or just maintain overall fitness? Knowing your goals will help you determine the type of equipment that will best suit your needs.

Take a moment to think about your specific objectives. For example, if your main goal is to lose weight and improve overall fitness, you might want a mix of cardio and strength training equipment. If you're focused on building muscle, strength training gear will be your priority. Clear goals will make your equipment choices much easier.

Selecting Cardio Machines

Cardiovascular exercise is vital for heart health, increasing endurance, and burning calories. There are various types of cardio machines to consider for your home gym, such as treadmills, ellipticals, stationary bikes, and rowing machines.

- Treadmills: If you enjoy walking or running, a treadmill might be a suitable option. Look for one with adjustable incline settings and cushioned decks for added comfort. A treadmill can be great for a range of cardio workouts, from brisk walks to intense runs.
- Ellipticals: Elliptical machines provide a low-impact workout that's easy on the joints. They offer a full-body workout, targeting both the upper and lower body. This can be a great option if you're looking for a less strenuous form of cardio.

- Stationary Bikes: These are ideal for those who prefer seated workouts. Stationary bikes focus on lower body strength and cardiovascular health. You can choose between upright bikes and recumbent bikes based on your comfort preference.
- Rowing Machines: Rowing machines provide a fantastic full-body workout, engaging major muscle groups while also improving cardiovascular fitness. They're great for both strength and cardio, making them a versatile choice.

When choosing a cardio machine, consider the space available in your home gym and select one that aligns with your fitness goals and preferences.

Choosing Strength Training Equipment

Strength training is crucial for building muscle, increasing bone density, and improving overall strength and stability. Here are some common types of strength training equipment to consider:

- Free Weights: Dumbbells and barbells offer versatility and can be used for a wide range of exercises. They're perfect for both beginners and advanced lifters. Adjustable dumbbells can save space and money by combining multiple weights into one set.

- Weight Machines: These provide stability and support, making them suitable for beginners or those who prefer guided movements. They can be a bit bulkier, so ensure you have enough space.
- Resistance Bands: Compact, portable, and perfect for adding resistance to bodyweight exercises. They're an excellent option for those with limited space.
- Suspension Trainers (like TRX): These utilize bodyweight and leverage to build strength and stability. They're versatile and take up very little space, making them ideal for small home gyms.

When selecting strength training equipment, consider the range of exercises you can perform with each piece and how it fits into your overall fitness routine.

Exploring Accessories

Accessories can enhance your workout experience and add variety to your routines. Here are some accessories to consider for your home gym:

- Stability Balls: Great for core exercises, stretching, and improving balance.
- Foam Rollers: Excellent for self-myofascial release, helping to alleviate muscle tension and improve mobility.
- Yoga Mats: Provide cushioning and grip for yoga or floor-based exercises.
- Medicine Balls: Useful for functional training exercises, focusing on strength, power, and explosive movements.

Consider your specific workout needs and available space when selecting accessories.

Choosing Based on Space and Budget Constraints

When selecting equipment for your home gym, it's essential to consider your available space and budget constraints:

- Measure Your Space: Measure the dimensions of your workout area and account for additional space needed for equipment movement and clearance. This will help you avoid purchasing equipment that doesn't fit comfortably.

- Set a Budget: Determine your budget and prioritize essential equipment based on your fitness goals. Research different brands, compare prices, and read reviews to ensure you're getting the best value for your money.
- Long-term Costs: Consider the long-term costs of maintenance, repairs, and potential upgrades. Investing in high-quality equipment can save money in the long run by reducing these additional costs.
- DIY Options and Alternatives: If you have limited space or a tight budget, consider alternatives like resistance bands or bodyweight exercises. Adjustable dumbbells, for example, can save space and costs compared to a full set of fixed weights.

Consulting with fitness professionals or trainers can offer valuable guidance in choosing the right equipment based on your individual needs and goals. Remember, the equipment you select should align with your fitness goals, fit comfortably within your available space, and be within your budget.

By choosing the right equipment, you can create a home gym that meets your needs and supports your journey towards fitness and well-being.

Chapter 5: Creating a Functional Workout Space

Now that we've covered selecting the right equipment, let's move on to creating a functional workout space. This chapter is all about organizing your equipment and finding storage solutions to maximize efficiency and convenience in your home gym. We'll also explore multi-functional and space-saving equipment options to make the most of your available space. Let's dive in!

Organizing Equipment

Efficiently organizing your workout equipment is crucial for creating a functional and enjoyable workout space. Here are some tips to help you optimize your equipment organization:

Categorize and Group Equipment:

1. Start by categorizing your equipment based on their usage and purpose. Group similar items together, such as cardio machines, free weights, resistance bands, and accessories. This way, you'll have a clear idea of where

everything is and can easily locate and access the equipment you need during your workouts.

Utilize Storage Solutions:

2. Invest in storage solutions that can effectively accommodate and organize your equipment. Wall-mounted racks, shelves, and cabinets are excellent options for keeping your equipment off the floor and creating a clutter-free environment. Choose storage solutions that are sturdy and durable enough to hold the weight of your equipment. For instance, you could use a wall-mounted rack for your free weights and resistance bands, and a cabinet with adjustable shelves for smaller accessories like yoga mats and foam rollers.

Consider Accessibility:

3. Arrange your equipment in a way that allows for easy access. Place frequently used items within reach and keep less frequently used equipment towards the

back or on higher shelves. This will save you time and effort during your workouts and ensure that you stay motivated. For example, keep your most-used dumbbells and resistance bands on a lower shelf or rack where you can easily grab them.

Space-Saving Equipment Options

When space is limited, selecting equipment that offers multiple functions and takes up minimal space is key. Here are some ideas for incorporating multi-functional and space-saving equipment in your home gym:

Adjustable Dumbbells:

1. Investing in a set of adjustable dumbbells can save you a considerable amount of space. These dumbbells allow you to change the weight settings easily, eliminating the need for multiple sets of dumbbells. They're versatile and can be used for various exercises, including upper body and lower body workouts. Imagine having a single set of dumbbells that can adjust from 5

pounds to 50 pounds—perfect for a variety of exercises without the clutter.

Resistance Bands:

2. Resistance bands are lightweight, portable, and highly versatile. They can be used to target different muscle groups and provide varying levels of resistance. Resistance bands are an excellent alternative to bulky weight machines and take up minimal space in your home gym. You can easily store them in a drawer or hang them on a wall-mounted hook.

Suspension Trainers:

3. Suspension trainers, like TRX, offer a full-body workout using just a single piece of equipment. They can be attached to a doorframe, overhead beam, or wall anchor and provide resistance and stability training. Suspension trainers are compact and can be easily stored when not in use. With suspension trainers, you can perform a wide range of exercises, from

pull-ups to core workouts, all with one piece of equipment.

Foldable Cardio Equipment:

4. If you're tight on space, consider investing in foldable cardio equipment. Foldable treadmills, ellipticals, and exercise bikes allow you to easily store them in a corner or under a bed when not in use. This way, you can have the cardio equipment you need without sacrificing space when you're not working out.

Wall-Mounted Pull-Up Bars:

5. A wall-mounted pull-up bar is an excellent space-saving option for upper body strength training. These bars can be easily installed on any sturdy wall and provide a challenging and effective workout. Additionally, some wall-mounted pull-up bars can double as suspension trainers for added versatility. This means you can do pull-ups, chin-ups, and use it for suspension training exercises, all with one installation.

By organizing your equipment effectively and incorporating multi-functional and space-saving options, you can create a functional workout space even in a limited area. This will not only enhance the efficiency of your workouts but also make your home gym more enjoyable and motivating.

Chapter 6: Personalizing Your Environment

Now that we've organized your equipment and designed a functional workout space, it's time to add some personal touches. Personalizing your home gym can make a huge difference in your motivation and overall workout experience. In this chapter, we'll explore strategies for enhancing the ambiance of your gym through decor, lighting, and motivational elements. Let's dive in and make your gym space uniquely yours!

Enhancing the Ambiance with Decor

Decorating your home gym can be a fun and creative process. It's an opportunity to reflect your personality and fitness journey. Here are some tips to help you personalize your gym space:

Choose an Inspirational Theme:

1. Consider selecting a theme that resonates with your fitness goals and interests. Whether it's a minimalist style, a sports-themed gym, or a nature-inspired oasis, aligning your decor with

a specific theme can create a cohesive and motivating environment. Think about what inspires you—maybe it's sleek, modern lines or a more rustic, natural feel.

Display Motivational Posters or Wall Art:

2. Hang up motivational posters or wall art that feature inspirational quotes, images of your favorite athletes, or depictions of nature. These visuals will serve as constant reminders of your dedication and provide the extra push you need during your workouts. You can even create a gallery wall with a mix of quotes and images that inspire you.

Incorporate Mirrors:

3. Mirrors are not only practical for checking your form during exercises but also add depth and brightness to your gym space. They can create an illusion of a larger area and reflect natural light, making your home gym feel brighter and more inviting. Plus, seeing your

progress in the mirror can be a great motivator!

Lighting for a Positive Atmosphere

Proper lighting is crucial for setting the right mood and ambiance in your home gym. Here are some tips to optimize lighting in your space:

Natural Light:

1. If possible, position your gym near windows or in a room with ample natural light. Natural light not only improves visibility but also boosts mood and energy levels, making your workouts more enjoyable. If your space allows, consider sheer curtains that let in plenty of light while maintaining privacy.

Artificial Lighting Options:

2. Ensure adequate artificial lighting for your home gym, especially if natural light is limited. Consider a combination of ceiling lights, adjustable track lighting, or strategically placed floor lamps.

Experiment with different lighting levels to find what works best for you. For example, overhead lights can be complemented with floor lamps that provide targeted lighting for specific workout areas.

Dimmable Lighting:

3. Install dimmable lighting fixtures to create a more versatile atmosphere. Dimming the lights during stretching or yoga sessions can create a calming and relaxing mood, while brightening them during high-intensity workouts can increase energy levels. Dimmable lights give you control over the ambiance depending on the type of workout you're doing.

Color Temperature:

4. Pay attention to the color temperature of your lighting. Opt for daylight or cool white bulbs (5000K-6500K) as they mimic natural sunlight and create a vibrant and energetic atmosphere. Avoid warm white bulbs (2700K-3000K) as

they can make the space feel cozy and potentially decrease motivation. The right lighting can make your gym feel more professional and motivating.

Motivational Elements

To further personalize your home gym and boost motivation, consider incorporating these elements:

Music:

1. Set up a speaker system or use wireless headphones to play your favorite workout music. Music can energize and motivate you during your workouts, making them more enjoyable and helping you push through challenging moments. Create playlists that match the intensity of your workouts, whether it's high-energy beats for cardio or calming tunes for yoga.

Inspirational Quotes and Affirmations:

2. Write down your favorite inspirational quotes or affirmations on a whiteboard

or chalkboard and place it in your gym space. Seeing these positive messages can encourage you to stay focused and push yourself further. You can change these messages regularly to keep things fresh and inspiring.

Display Goals and Progress:

3. Visualize your fitness goals by creating a vision board or displaying a calendar to track your progress. Seeing the milestones you've achieved and the work you've put in can be highly motivating and remind you of why you started this journey. A bulletin board or a digital display can serve as a constant reminder of your progress and goals.

By personalizing your home gym environment through decor, lighting, and motivational elements, you can create a positive and energizing atmosphere that enhances your workout experience. Take the time to design a space that reflects your personality, goals, and interests, ensuring that your home gym becomes your sanctuary for achieving fitness success.

Chapter 7: Safety and Maintenance

Now that your home gym is coming together, it's time to focus on something super important: safety and maintenance. Ensuring the safety of your home gym is crucial to prevent accidents and injuries during your workouts. Let's dive into how you can keep your gym safe and your equipment in top shape.

Importance of Safety Considerations

Your home gym should be a place where you can work out confidently, knowing that you're safe from accidents and injuries. By following proper safety measures, you can ensure a secure workout environment. Here are some key considerations for maintaining a safe home gym:

Proper Equipment Assembly

When setting up your home gym, it's crucial to carefully read and follow the instructions for assembling your equipment. Improper assembly can lead to unstable structures or malfunctioning equipment, increasing the risk of accidents. Take your time to double-check that all components are securely fastened and in good working condition. If a manual seems unclear, look up instructional videos online or contact the manufacturer for assistance. Proper assembly is the first step to ensuring your equipment is safe to use.

Maintenance and Inspection

Regular maintenance and inspection of your home gym equipment are essential for both the longevity of the equipment and the safety of its users. Set up a routine to inspect your equipment for any signs of wear or damage, such as frayed cables, loose bolts, or worn-out parts. Address any issues promptly by repairing or replacing damaged equipment. This proactive approach will help you avoid accidents and keep your equipment running smoothly.

Injury Prevention

Preventing injuries should be a top priority in your home gym. Here are some important guidelines to keep in mind:

- Warm Up Properly: Before each workout, take time to warm up properly. This prepares your body for physical exertion and reduces the risk of injury.

- Use Proper Form and Technique: Always use proper form and technique when performing exercises to avoid strain or injury. If you're unsure about the correct form, consider consulting a trainer or watching instructional videos.
- Start Light: Begin with lighter weights or resistance and gradually increase the intensity as your strength and endurance improve.
- Use Safety Features: Always use safety features such as safety bars or spotter arms when using heavy weights or performing exercises that involve a risk of falling.
- Secure Resistance Bands and Cables: Ensure resistance bands or cables are securely anchored and inspect them regularly for signs of wear.
- Keep Your Workout Area Clean: Maintain a clean and clutter-free workout area to prevent tripping hazards. A tidy gym is a safe gym!

Establishing a Maintenance Routine

To ensure the longevity of your equipment and the safety of your workouts, it's essential to establish a regular maintenance routine. Here are some steps to include in your routine:

1. Clean Your Equipment: Regularly wipe down your equipment to remove sweat, dirt, and bacteria. Use a mild detergent and a damp cloth, and avoid harsh chemicals that may damage the equipment.
2. Lubricate Moving Parts: Check your equipment's instruction manual for any recommended lubrication points. Apply a suitable lubricant to keep the moving parts functioning smoothly.
3. Inspect Cables and Pulleys: Examine the cables and pulleys for any signs of wear, fraying, or damage. Replace any damaged cables immediately to prevent accidents.
4. Tighten Bolts and Screws: Periodically check all bolts and screws on your equipment to ensure they are securely tightened. Loose hardware can compromise the stability and safety of the equipment.
5. Check Weight Stacks: If you have weight stacks in your home gym equipment, inspect them regularly for proper alignment and secure

attachment. Make sure the weight pins are fully inserted, and there are no loose plates.

6. Test Safety Features: Ensure that all safety features, such as locking pins, safety bars, and emergency stop buttons, are functioning correctly. Test them periodically to confirm that they provide the necessary protection.

Creating a Safe and Enjoyable Workout Environment

By following these maintenance practices and safety guidelines, you can create a safe and enjoyable workout environment in your home gym. Stay diligent in your maintenance routine to keep your equipment in optimal condition and to prevent accidents or injuries during your workouts.

Regularly maintaining your gym equipment not only ensures your safety but also extends the life of your investments. It might seem like a hassle, but a few minutes spent on maintenance each week can save you a lot of trouble down the line.

Chapter 8: Maximizing Workouts

Now that your home gym is set up and safe, it's time to talk about maximizing your workouts. This chapter is all about making the most of your equipment and space by designing versatile workouts and incorporating variety and progression. These strategies will help you prevent plateaus and keep your motivation high. Let's dive in!

Designing Versatile Workouts

Designing versatile workouts allows you to make the most of your home gym and the equipment you have. Here are some techniques to help you achieve this:

Circuit Training:

1. Circuit training involves moving through a series of exercises with minimal rest in between. This allows you to target different muscle groups while keeping your heart rate elevated. For example, you might start with a set of squats, move on to push-ups, then do some bent-over rows, and finish with planks. By strategically incorporating various

exercises using different equipment, you can create a versatile workout that engages your entire body. This method is great for both strength and cardio, making your workouts efficient and effective.

Superset and Tri-set Training:

2. Superset and tri-set training involve performing exercises back-to-back with little to no rest in between. A superset typically includes two exercises, while a tri-set includes three. This technique allows you to target specific muscle groups while maximizing your time and effort. For instance, you could pair a chest press with a row for a superset, targeting both the front and back of your upper body. Tri-sets could include a leg press, calf raise, and leg curl, giving your lower body a comprehensive workout. By combining exercises that complement each other, you can create an efficient and effective workout routine.

Interval Training:

3. Interval training involves alternating between periods of high-intensity exercise and periods of rest or lower intensity. This type of workout is particularly effective for cardiovascular conditioning and can be adapted for various forms of cardio equipment, such as treadmills, stationary bikes, or rowing machines. For example, you might sprint for 30 seconds on a treadmill, then walk for a minute, and repeat. By adjusting the duration and intensity of your intervals, you can create a challenging and versatile workout routine that boosts your endurance and burns calories.

Functional Training:

4. Functional training focuses on movements that mimic daily activities and improve overall strength, balance, and coordination. By incorporating functional exercises into your workout routine, such as squats, lunges, and planks, you can enhance your overall fitness and make your workouts more practical and applicable to real-life

activities. For example, practicing squats can help improve your ability to lift objects from the ground safely.

Incorporating Variety and Progression

To prevent plateaus and maintain motivation, it's important to incorporate variety and progression into your workout routines. Here are some ideas to help you achieve this:

Exercise Variation:

1. Instead of sticking to the same exercises every time, try incorporating different variations or alternatives to target the same muscle groups. For example, instead of always doing traditional bicep curls, you can switch to hammer curls or concentration curls. This not only keeps your workouts interesting but also challenges your muscles in new ways. Mixing up your routine helps prevent boredom and keeps your muscles guessing.

Different Training Modalities:

2. In addition to traditional weightlifting exercises, consider incorporating other training modalities into your workout routine. This can include bodyweight exercises, yoga or Pilates, resistance band workouts, or high-intensity interval training (HIIT). By diversifying your training methods, you can engage different muscle groups and work on different aspects of fitness. For instance, a weekly routine might include weightlifting on Monday, yoga on Wednesday, and HIIT on Friday, giving you a well-rounded fitness regimen.

Progression Strategies:

3. To continue making progress and pushing yourself, it's important to gradually increase the intensity or difficulty of your workouts. Some progression strategies include increasing the weight or resistance, adding more repetitions or sets, reducing rest periods, or incorporating advanced variations of exercises. For example, if you've been doing three sets of 10 push-ups, try adding a fourth set

or switching to decline push-ups. By progressively challenging yourself, you can continue to see improvements and stay motivated.

By designing versatile workouts and incorporating variety and progression, you can maximize the effectiveness of your home gym and keep your fitness journey exciting and rewarding. Experiment with different techniques and find what works best for you. Remember, the key is to keep your workouts dynamic and challenging.

Chapter 9: Integrating Technology

In today's digital age, technology is everywhere, and it's become an integral part of our fitness routines as well. Integrating technology into your home gym can offer a wide range of benefits, from tracking your progress to staying motivated. In this chapter, we'll explore various technology options that can enhance your home gym experience and provide tips on seamlessly incorporating them into your workout routine. Let's get started!

Exploring Technology Options

Fitness Apps:

1. Fitness apps have exploded in popularity because they offer a convenient way to track workouts, set goals, and monitor progress. There are countless fitness apps available, catering to different fitness levels and goals. These apps often provide workout plans, exercise tutorials, and the ability to track metrics like calories burned, distance covered, and heart rate. Imagine having a virtual trainer right at your fingertips, guiding you

through workouts and helping you stay on track. Popular apps include MyFitnessPal, Strava, and Nike Training Club.

Virtual Trainers:

2. Virtual trainers are another technological advancement that can significantly enhance your home gym experience. These trainers provide personalized workout plans based on your goals and fitness level. They can offer real-time feedback, correct your form, and motivate you during workouts. Virtual trainers simulate the experience of working with a personal trainer, providing guidance and encouragement to help you achieve your fitness goals. Platforms like Peloton and Mirror offer interactive training sessions that can make you feel like you're in a live class.

Interactive Equipment Features:

3. Many modern fitness equipment models come equipped with interactive features. These might include touchscreens with built-in workout programs, video demonstrations, and virtual training

sessions. Some equipment also integrates with fitness apps and wearable devices, allowing you to track your progress and sync data seamlessly. These interactive features can add excitement and engagement to your workouts, making them more enjoyable and effective. Brands like NordicTrack and ProForm offer equipment with such advanced features.

Tips for Integrating Technology

Assess Your Needs:

1. Before diving into the world of fitness technology, assess your specific needs and goals. Consider what areas of your fitness routine could benefit from technology—whether it's tracking your progress, accessing workout programs, or receiving real-time feedback. Understanding your needs will help you narrow down the technology options that align with your goals. For instance, if you're looking to improve your running, a fitness app with detailed running analytics might be best for you.

Research and Test:

2. Take the time to research different technology options and read reviews from reputable sources. Look for features that match your needs and budget. Additionally, many fitness apps and virtual trainers offer free trials—take advantage of these to test out different options before committing to a long-term subscription. Trying out a few different apps or virtual trainers can help you find the one that fits your style and preferences.

Create a Seamless Integration:

3. Once you've chosen the technology you want to integrate into your home gym, set it up in a way that seamlessly fits into your workout routine. This could involve syncing your fitness app with your wearable device or setting up your virtual trainer on a tablet or TV screen. Organize your technology so it's easily accessible during your workouts, ensuring it enhances rather than disrupts your routine. For example, mount a tablet holder on your exercise bike for easy access to virtual classes.

Utilize Data and Progress Tracking:

4. Take advantage of the data and progress tracking features offered by fitness apps and wearable devices. Set goals, track your workouts, and monitor your progress over time. This can provide valuable insights into your performance, helping you identify areas for improvement and stay motivated. Reviewing your progress regularly can also help you celebrate your achievements and adjust your goals as needed.

Embrace Variety:

5. Technology can open up a world of workout possibilities. Experiment with different workout programs and classes offered through fitness apps or virtual trainers. This variety can prevent boredom and plateaus, keeping your workouts challenging and exciting. For example, mix up your routine with yoga, HIIT, and strength training classes available through your app or virtual trainer.

Stay Motivated:

6. Use the motivational features of fitness apps and virtual trainers to your advantage. Set reminders for your workouts, participate in challenges or competitions, and leverage the community aspect of these platforms. Surround yourself with like-minded individuals who can support and motivate you on your fitness journey. Many apps offer community features where you can join groups, share your progress, and get encouragement from others.

Integrating technology into your home gym can greatly enhance your workout experience. Whether you're using fitness apps to track your progress or virtual trainers to guide your workouts, technology offers numerous benefits for motivation, progress tracking, and personalized training. Embrace these technological advancements and let them take your home gym workouts to the next level.

Chapter 10: Staying Consistent and Adapting

We're almost at the finish line in our journey to building and maintaining the perfect home gym. In this chapter, we'll dive into strategies for staying consistent with your workouts and adapting your routine over time. Consistency is key to achieving your fitness goals, and it can be tough to maintain a regular workout schedule. We'll explore how to establish a sustainable routine, overcome common challenges like motivation slumps and time constraints, and adapt your home gym setup and workouts as your needs change. Let's get started!

Establishing a Sustainable Workout Routine

The first step towards staying consistent is creating a workout schedule and sticking to it. Treat your workout sessions like important appointments that you can't miss. Set specific days and times for your workouts, and make them a priority in your daily routine. Here are some tips to help you establish a sustainable workout routine:

Create a Schedule:

1. Choose specific days and times for your workouts. Whether it's early mornings, during lunch breaks, or evenings, find what works best for you and stick to it. Consistency will help you build the habit of exercising regularly.

Find Enjoyable Activities:

2. It's easier to stay motivated when you genuinely enjoy the exercise you're doing. Experiment with different types of workouts, such as cardio, strength training, and flexibility exercises, to find what resonates with you. If you're having fun during your workouts, you'll be more likely to stick with them in the long run.

Build Accountability:

3. Accountability is crucial for maintaining a consistent workout routine. Consider finding a workout buddy or joining a fitness group or class. Having someone

to exercise with can provide motivation and support, as well as make the workouts more enjoyable. You can also set goals together and track each other's progress, increasing accountability and commitment.

Overcoming Common Challenges

Motivation slumps and time constraints are common obstacles that can hinder your consistency. Here's how to overcome them:

Motivation Slumps:

1. To overcome motivation slumps, find ways to stay inspired. Set short-term and long-term goals that are specific, measurable, attainable, relevant, and time-bound (SMART goals). Tracking your progress towards these goals and celebrating your achievements will help you stay motivated.
    - Vary Your Workouts: Incorporate different exercises, change the order of your routine, or try new fitness classes. By adding variety, you can keep your workouts fresh and exciting,

preventing boredom and
maintaining motivation.

Time Constraints:

2. Even with busy schedules, it's possible
   to find pockets of time for exercise.
   Break your workouts into shorter, more
   manageable sessions throughout the
   day if necessary. Wake up a little earlier,
   make use of lunch breaks, or allocate
   specific time slots for exercise in the
   evening. Consistency in small
   increments is still progress.

Adapting the Home Gym Setup and Workout Routine

As your fitness goals and lifestyle evolve, it's
important to adapt your home gym setup and
workout routine accordingly. Here's how to do
it:

Regularly Assess Your Goals:

1. Regularly assess your fitness goals and
   make adjustments to ensure they

remain aligned with your priorities. Consider consulting with fitness professionals or trainers to receive guidance on modifying your workout program and equipment choices.

Evaluate Your Space and Equipment:

2. Regularly evaluate your available space and equipment. If you find that you're not using certain equipment or if you need to make room for new additions, consider selling or donating unused items. This will declutter your space and make it more functional for your current needs.

Embrace Variety:

3. Explore new workout techniques or classes that align with your evolving goals. Incorporate different training modalities to challenge your body in various ways and prevent plateaus. Stay up-to-date with fitness trends and research to ensure you're continually challenging yourself and enjoying your workouts.

Building a Routine that Adapts to Life

Your life isn't static, and neither should your workout routine be. Here are some additional tips for building a flexible routine that adapts to your changing life:

Set Flexible Goals:

1. Set both long-term and short-term goals that can adapt to changes in your life. For instance, if you're preparing for a big event, your goals might shift towards more intense training. After the event, you might focus on recovery and maintenance.

Listen to Your Body:

2. Pay attention to how your body feels and be willing to adjust your workouts accordingly. If you're feeling fatigued or experiencing pain, it might be time to scale back and focus on recovery.

Plan for Breaks:

3. Life happens, and sometimes you need a break from your routine. Whether it's a vacation, a busy work period, or recovering from an illness, plan for these breaks and have a strategy to get back on track.

Celebrate Small Wins:

4. Consistency isn't about being perfect; it's about making progress. Celebrate your small wins and recognize that every step forward is a success.

By establishing a sustainable workout routine, overcoming common challenges, and being open to change, you can achieve long-term fitness success. Keep pushing yourself, stay motivated, and remember that your home gym is a flexible and personalized space that can evolve with you and your goals.

Conclusion

As we conclude "Home Gym Mastery: Building Your Perfect Workout Space," it's clear that creating an effective and enjoyable home gym is a rewarding endeavor that can significantly enhance your fitness journey. Throughout this book, we've explored the essential steps to assess your space, set achievable goals, design an efficient layout, select appropriate equipment, and create a personalized and functional workout environment.

Remember, the key to a successful home gym lies in thoughtful planning and continuous adaptation. Stay informed about the latest fitness trends, be open to modifying your space and routine as your needs evolve, and always prioritize safety and maintenance. By implementing the strategies and insights shared in this book, you'll be well-equipped to build and maintain a home gym that keeps you motivated and supports your fitness goals.

Made in United States
Troutdale, OR
09/20/2024

22996645R00037